MW01168959

Nuts and Seeds Guide for Beginners

Importance of Nuts and Seeds in Nutrition

By

Cedric Macallister
Copyright@2023

Table of Contents

CHAPTER 1

Introduction to Nuts and Seeds

1.1 What are Nuts and Seeds?

The classification of nuts and seeds is a fascinating exploration into the diverse world of plant-based foods and their botanical structures.

Understanding Nuts and Seeds

1. Definition and Botanical Distinctions:

Nuts and seeds are foundational components of plants, vital for reproduction and propagation. While often used interchangeably, they possess distinct botanical identities.

- **Nuts:** Botanically, nuts are hard-shelled fruits that encapsulate seeds. These seeds are typically enclosed within a tough, indehiscent (non-splitting) shell that protects them. Examples include acorns, chestnuts, and hazelnuts.

- **Seeds:** Seeds, on the other hand, are the reproductive units of flowering plants. They can be found within the fruits of these plants and come in various sizes, shapes, and textures. They can be encased within fleshy fruits like apples or nestled in dry pods like those of sunflowers.

2. Diversity and Varieties:

- **Tree Nuts:** Derived from trees, these nuts grow within a hard outer shell. They include almonds, walnuts, pecans, cashews, and more. Each type boasts unique nutritional profiles and flavors.

- **Ground Nuts:** These nuts grow underground, encompassing peanuts and other leguminous seeds. They vary in taste, texture, and culinary applications.

- **Edible Seeds:** Seeds such as chia, flax, pumpkin, and sunflower seeds, despite not being nuts by botanical definition, offer remarkable nutritional benefits and culinary versatility.

3. Culinary Significance:

- **Rich Flavor Profiles:** Nuts and seeds contribute diverse flavors, from the buttery richness of almonds to the earthy crunch of pumpkin seeds. They add depth, texture, and taste to an array of dishes, ranging from savory to sweet.

- **Versatile Use:** These ingredients feature prominently in cuisines worldwide, being used whole, chopped, roasted, ground, or even as oils and spreads. They're integral to salads, baked goods, spreads, and main dishes, amplifying both taste and nutritional value.

4. Nutritional Powerhouses:

- **Nutrient Density:** Nuts and seeds are nutrient-dense, boasting healthy fats, proteins, vitamins, minerals, and antioxidants. They offer essential nutrients like omega-3 fatty acids, vitamin E, magnesium, and plant-based proteins, contributing to overall health and well-being.

5. Health Benefits:

- **Heart Health:** Regular consumption of nuts has been linked to reduced risks of heart disease due to their heart-friendly fats and compounds that help manage cholesterol levels.

- **Brain Function:** Omega-3-rich seeds like flax and chia seeds are known to support brain health and cognitive function.

- **Weight Management:** Contrary to common belief, incorporating nuts and seeds into a balanced diet may aid in

weight management due to
their satiating effect.

6. Cultural Significance:

- **Historical and Cultural
  Significance:** Nuts and seeds
  have been integral to human
  diets for centuries, holding
  cultural and symbolic
  importance in various traditions
  and cuisines worldwide.
  They've been used in rituals,
  ceremonies, and traditional
  medicines across diverse
  cultures.

In essence, nuts and seeds are not
only culinary delights but also
nutritional powerhouses with
historical, cultural, and botanical
significance. Their versatile nature
and health benefits make them
integral components of a balanced

diet and a source of exploration for food enthusiasts and health-conscious individuals alike.

1.2 Importance of Nuts and Seeds in Nutrition

The importance of nuts and seeds in nutrition is multifaceted and deeply rooted in their rich nutritional composition and health-promoting properties.

Nutritional Value:

1. Essential Nutrients:

- **Healthy Fats:** Nuts and seeds are abundant sources of healthy fats, including monounsaturated and polyunsaturated fats such as omega-3 and omega-6 fatty acids. These fats support heart health, brain function, and overall well-being.

- **Proteins:** They provide plant-based proteins, making them valuable alternatives for individuals following vegetarian or vegan diets.

- **Vitamins and Minerals:** Nuts and seeds contain an array of essential vitamins (such as vitamin E, B vitamins) and minerals (such as magnesium, zinc, and calcium) crucial for various bodily functions, including immune support, bone health, and energy metabolism.

2. Antioxidants and Phytochemicals:

- **Antioxidants:** Rich in antioxidants like vitamin E, selenium, and various polyphenols, nuts and seeds combat oxidative stress, reduce inflammation, and contribute to cell health and longevity.

- **Phytochemicals:** These bioactive compounds present in nuts and seeds have shown potential health benefits, including anti-cancer properties, immune support, and cardiovascular health promotion.

Health Benefits:

1. Heart Health:

- **Reduced Risk of Cardiovascular Diseases:** Regular consumption of nuts, particularly almonds, walnuts, and pistachios, has been associated with lowered risks of heart disease due to their ability to reduce LDL cholesterol and improve overall lipid profiles.

2. Weight Management:

- **Satiety and Weight Control:** Despite being calorie-dense, nuts and seeds have a high satiety value, leading to reduced overall calorie intake. Incorporating moderate amounts into a diet may actually aid in weight management.

3. Brain Health:

- **Omega-3 Fatty Acids:** Seeds like flaxseeds and chia seeds, as well as walnuts, are rich in omega-3 fatty acids known to support brain health, cognitive function, and potentially reduce the risk of neurodegenerative diseases.

4. Diabetes Management:

- **Blood Sugar Control:** Certain nuts and seeds, like almonds and chia seeds, have been linked to improved blood sugar control due to their fiber content and beneficial effects on insulin sensitivity.

Versatility in Culinary Use:

1. Diverse Applications:

- **Culinary Flexibility:** Nuts and seeds add texture, flavor, and nutritional value to an extensive range of dishes, including salads, stir-fries, baked goods, and smoothies. They're versatile ingredients that can be used whole, chopped, ground, or turned into spreads and oils.

2. Substitution and Inclusion:

- **Substituting Unhealthy Ingredients:** Nuts and seeds often serve as healthier substitutes for processed snacks, animal-based proteins, and refined oils, contributing to a more balanced and nutrient-rich diet.

nuts and seeds play a pivotal role in enhancing nutritional intake, providing essential nutrients, promoting health, and offering culinary diversity. Their inclusion in a balanced diet contributes significantly to overall well-being, making them a valuable and versatile addition to everyday meals and dietary choices.

1.3 Culinary and Cultural Significance

The culinary and cultural significance of nuts and seeds spans centuries, influencing cuisines worldwide and holding symbolic importance in various cultures.

Culinary Significance:

1. Flavor Enhancement:

- **Texture and Taste:** Nuts and seeds offer diverse textures, from creamy to crunchy, and a wide range of flavors, including nutty, earthy, and sometimes sweet or savory notes. They contribute depth and richness to dishes, elevating both taste and visual appeal.

2. Versatile Use in Cooking:

- **Ingredient Diversity:** Nuts and seeds are used across culinary traditions in both sweet and savory dishes. They're incorporated in salads, stir-fries, curries, pastries, sauces, and desserts, showcasing their adaptability and ability to complement various cuisines.

3. Culinary Techniques:

- **Roasting and Grinding:** Roasting intensifies their flavors, while grinding them into pastes or flours enhances their versatility, allowing for use in spreads, coatings, and baking.

4. Nut and Seed Oils:

- **Nutritional Oils:** Extracted oils from nuts and seeds, like almond oil, sesame oil, and sunflower seed oil, not only add distinctive flavors but also serve as healthy alternatives for cooking and dressings.

Cultural Significance:

1. Traditional Cuisine:

- **Integral in Cultural Dishes:** Nuts and seeds hold a prominent place in traditional cuisines worldwide. For example:

  - In Middle Eastern cuisine, dishes like hummus (made from chickpeas and sesame seeds) and baklava (layered pastry with nuts and honey) showcase their importance.

- In Asian cuisines, sesame seeds, peanuts, and cashews are frequently used in various dishes, from stir-fries to desserts.

- Latin American cuisine incorporates seeds like pumpkin and chia in beverages, baked goods, and savory dishes.

2. Symbolism and Rituals:

- **Symbolic Significance:** Nuts and seeds often hold symbolic meanings in cultural practices and rituals. They might symbolize fertility, prosperity, or be used in ceremonies and traditional medicine.

3. Festivals and Celebrations:

- **Incorporated in Festive Foods:** Many cultural celebrations and festivals feature dishes where nuts and seeds play a central role. These dishes often have historical and ceremonial significance, showcasing the cultural value attached to these ingredients.

Health and Cultural Fusion:

- **Health-Conscious Adaptation:** As people embrace healthier eating habits, traditional dishes incorporating nuts and seeds are being reimagined to align with modern health-conscious choices. For instance, traditional desserts are being revamped using healthier alternatives like almond flour or incorporating seeds for added nutritional value.

The culinary and cultural significance of nuts and seeds goes beyond their taste and nutritional value. They're intertwined with cultural heritage, traditional practices, and culinary creativity, serving as a bridge between heritage-rich cuisines and modern health-conscious adaptations. Their diverse applications and symbolic significance continue to shape culinary experiences and cultural identities globally.

CHAPTER 2

Types of Nuts

2.1 Tree Nuts

2.1.1 Almonds

- **Botanical Profile:** Almonds belong to the Prunus genus and are classified as drupes, characterized by a hard outer shell encasing a single seed or kernel.

- **Nutritional Highlights:** Almonds are nutrient powerhouses, rich in healthy fats, protein, fiber, vitamin E, magnesium, and antioxidants. They are renowned for their heart-healthy properties and are a source of plant-based proteins.

- **Culinary Uses:** Almonds are incredibly versatile, used in various forms—whole, sliced, chopped, ground, or as almond butter or almond milk. They feature prominently in both sweet and savory dishes, from salads and stir-fries to pastries and desserts.

2.1.2 Walnuts

- **Botanical Profile:** Walnuts are seeds of drupe fruits belonging to the Juglans genus. They have a wrinkled, hard shell that encases two bumpy lobes.

- **Nutritional Highlights:** Walnuts are rich in omega-3 fatty acids, antioxidants, protein, fiber, vitamin E, and several minerals like copper and manganese. Their omega-3 content contributes to heart health and cognitive function.

- **Culinary Uses:** Walnuts have a distinct flavor and texture, making them popular in baking, salads, pestos, and as a topping for yogurt or oatmeal. Walnut oil is also prized for its flavor and used in dressings and cooking.

2.1.3 Pecans

- **Botanical Profile:** Pecans are drupes that belong to the Carya genus. They have a smooth, oblong shell that splits easily to reveal two halves.

- **Nutritional Highlights:** Pecans are rich in monounsaturated fats, antioxidants, fiber, vitamins (like vitamin E and B vitamins), and minerals (such as manganese and zinc). They are known for their heart-healthy benefits and contribute to improved digestion.

- **Culinary Uses:** Pecans have a buttery, rich flavor, making them a staple in desserts like pecan pie. They're also used in salads, savory dishes, and as a topping for breakfast foods.

2.1.4 Cashews

- **Botanical Profile:** Cashews come from the Anacardium genus and are seeds found at the bottom of the cashew apple. They have a distinctive kidney-shaped shell.

- **Nutritional Highlights:** Cashews are lower in fat

compared to many other nuts but contain healthy monounsaturated fats. They are a good source of protein, minerals like copper and magnesium, and vitamins like B6 and K.

- **Culinary Uses:** Cashews have a creamy texture when blended, making them ideal for dairy-free alternatives like cashew cream or as a base for sauces and vegan cheeses. They're also enjoyed roasted as snacks and used in various cuisines, especially Asian dishes.

2.1.5 Brazil Nuts

- **Botanical Profile:** Brazil nuts are seeds from the Bertholletia excelsa tree. They are enclosed in a hard, round shell that contains several seeds within.

- **Nutritional Highlights:** Brazil nuts are notable for their high selenium content, providing a substantial amount of this essential mineral in just a few nuts. They also contain healthy fats, protein, and other nutrients.

- **Culinary Uses:** Brazil nuts have a rich, creamy flavor and are often eaten raw or roasted as snacks. They're also chopped and added to desserts, used in nut mixes, or ground into flour for baking.

Tree nuts, including almonds, walnuts, pecans, cashews, and Brazil nuts, offer a diverse array of flavors, textures, and nutritional benefits.

Their culinary versatility makes them invaluable in various cuisines and dietary preferences, while their rich nutrient profiles contribute significantly to overall health and well-being. Incorporating these nuts into a balanced diet adds depth, taste, and essential nutrients, making them an integral part of healthy eating habits.

2.2 Ground Nuts

2.2.1 Peanuts

- **Botanical Profile:** Peanuts, also known as groundnuts, are legumes that grow underground. They belong to the Arachis genus and are packed in a pod-like structure.

- **Nutritional Highlights:**
Peanuts are rich in protein,
healthy fats, fiber, vitamins
(like B vitamins), minerals
(such as magnesium and
phosphorus), and antioxidants
like resveratrol. They
contribute to heart health and
provide a substantial source of
plant-based proteins.

- **Culinary Uses:** Peanuts are
incredibly versatile and are
consumed in various forms—
roasted, boiled, as peanut
butter, oil, or used in sauces
like satay. They're central to
many cuisines worldwide, from
Asian stir-fries to peanut-based
African stews.

2.2.2 Hazelnuts

- **Botanical Profile:** Hazelnuts, also called filberts, come from the Corylus genus. They have a hard, spherical shell that encases the nut within.

- **Nutritional Highlights:** Hazelnuts are rich in healthy fats, particularly monounsaturated fats, and provide a good source of protein, fiber, vitamin E, manganese, and antioxidants. They promote heart health and contribute to skin health and collagen production.

- **Culinary Uses:** Hazelnuts have a distinct, slightly sweet flavor and are commonly used in confectionery, especially in chocolate spreads like Nutella. They're also utilized in baking, salads, and savory dishes, adding a rich, nutty flavor.

2.2.3 Chestnuts

- **Botanical Profile:** Chestnuts belong to the Castanea genus and have a hard outer shell with a prickly husk. They are unique among nuts as they have a higher starch content than fat.

- **Nutritional Highlights:** Chestnuts are lower in fat compared to other nuts but are a good source of complex carbohydrates, fiber, vitamins (such as vitamin C and B vitamins), and minerals like potassium and copper. They offer energy and contribute to immune health.

- **Culinary Uses:** Chestnuts have a sweet, creamy taste and are commonly roasted or boiled during the fall and winter seasons. They're used in stuffings, soups, desserts, and as purees in various cuisines worldwide.

2.2.4 Macadamia Nuts

- **Botanical Profile:** Macadamia nuts originate from the Macadamia genus and have an extremely hard shell, often considered the toughest nut to crack.

- **Nutritional Highlights:** Macadamia nuts are rich in monounsaturated fats, making them heart-healthy. They contain antioxidants, fiber, protein, vitamins (like vitamin B1 and B6), and minerals (such as magnesium and iron).

- **Culinary Uses:** Macadamia nuts have a creamy, buttery texture and a slightly sweet taste. They're enjoyed raw or roasted, used in baked goods, salads, and are popularly incorporated into desserts like cookies and cakes.

Ground nuts, including peanuts, hazelnuts, chestnuts, and macadamia nuts, offer a diverse range of flavors, textures, and nutritional benefits. From the protein-packed peanuts to the creamy richness of macadamia nuts, these varieties contribute significantly to global cuisines, offering culinary versatility and essential nutrients for a balanced diet.

CHAPTER 3

Varieties of Seeds

3.1 Edible Seeds

3.1.1 Chia Seeds

- **Botanical Profile:** Chia seeds come from the Salvia hispanica plant and were an essential part of ancient Mayan and Aztec diets. They are small, oval-shaped seeds that expand when exposed to liquid.

- **Nutritional Highlights:** Chia seeds are packed with fiber, omega-3 fatty acids, protein, antioxidants, vitamins (such as B vitamins), and minerals (like calcium and magnesium). They are renowned for promoting heart health, aiding digestion, and boosting energy.

- **Culinary Uses:** Chia seeds are incredibly versatile and are commonly used in puddings, smoothies, baked goods, and as a thickening agent in sauces or jams due to their gel-like consistency when soaked.

3.1.2 Flaxseeds

- **Botanical Profile:** Flaxseeds, derived from the Linum usitatissimum plant, have been cultivated for thousands of years and are among the oldest crops. They are small, flat seeds with a slightly nutty flavor.

- **Nutritional Highlights:** Flaxseeds are rich in omega-3 fatty acids, fiber, lignans (a type of antioxidant), protein, vitamins (like B vitamins), and minerals (such as manganese and magnesium). They support heart health, aid in digestion, and have potential anticancer properties.

- **Culinary Uses:** Ground flaxseeds are commonly used in baking as an egg substitute or added to smoothies, cereals, and yogurt. They can also be sprinkled over salads or incorporated into homemade granola bars.

3.1.3 Sunflower Seeds

- **Botanical Profile:** Sunflower seeds come from the Helianthus annuus plant and have been cultivated for centuries by indigenous cultures in the

Americas. They are small, elongated seeds found at the center of sunflower heads.

- **Nutritional Highlights:** Sunflower seeds are rich in healthy fats, protein, fiber, vitamins (such as vitamin E), minerals (like selenium and magnesium), and antioxidants. They promote heart health, aid in cell repair, and support skin health.

- **Culinary Uses:** Sunflower seeds are enjoyed roasted as a snack, used as toppings for salads or baked goods, or incorporated into trail mixes and granola. They're also pressed to extract sunflower oil for cooking.

3.1.4 Pumpkin Seeds (Pepitas)

- **Botanical Profile:** Pumpkin seeds, known as pepitas, come from various species of pumpkins and squash. They are flat, oval seeds found within the flesh of pumpkins.

- **Nutritional Highlights:** Pumpkin seeds are rich in protein, healthy fats, fiber, vitamins (such as vitamin E), minerals (like zinc and magnesium), and antioxidants. They support immune function, prostate health, and provide essential nutrients.

- **Culinary Uses:** Pumpkin seeds are enjoyed roasted as a snack, sprinkled over salads or soups, and used in baking, pesto, or as a crunchy topping for various dishes.

Edible seeds like chia seeds, flaxseeds, sunflower seeds, and pumpkin seeds offer an array of nutritional benefits and culinary versatility. Their rich nutrient profiles make them integral parts of balanced diets, while their adaptability in various recipes adds texture, flavor, and health benefits to a wide range of dishes.

3.2 Grain-like Seeds

3.2.1 Quinoa

- **Botanical Profile:** Quinoa, pronounced "keen-wah," is a pseudocereal from the Chenopodium quinoa plant. It's been cultivated for thousands of years in the Andes region and is known for its tiny, spherical seeds.

- **Nutritional Highlights:**
Quinoa is a complete protein, containing all nine essential amino acids. It's rich in fiber, vitamins (such as B vitamins), minerals (like magnesium and iron), antioxidants, and beneficial plant compounds. It supports heart health, aids in digestion, and provides sustained energy.

- **Culinary Uses:** Quinoa is incredibly versatile and used in salads, pilafs, soups, breakfast bowls, and as a substitute for rice or pasta. It comes in various colors like white, red, and black, offering different textures and flavors.

3.2.2 Amaranth

- **Botanical Profile:** Amaranth comes from the Amaranthus plant and has been cultivated for centuries by Aztecs and other Mesoamerican cultures. It's known for its tiny, grain-like seeds.

- **Nutritional Highlights:** Amaranth is rich in protein, fiber, vitamins (such as vitamin C and folate), minerals (like calcium and iron), and antioxidants like polyphenols. It aids in digestion, supports bone health, and may have anti-inflammatory properties.

- **Culinary Uses:** Amaranth seeds can be popped like popcorn or cooked into porridge, soups, and stews.

They're also used in baked goods like bread and incorporated into gluten-free flour blends.

3.2.3 Buckwheat

- **Botanical Profile:** Buckwheat comes from the Fagopyrum esculentum plant and is not botanically related to wheat. It's a pseudocereal known for its triangular seeds.

- **Nutritional Highlights:** Buckwheat is gluten-free and rich in protein, fiber, vitamins (like B vitamins), minerals (such as manganese and magnesium), antioxidants like rutin, and essential amino acids. It supports heart health, helps manage blood sugar levels, and aids digestion.

- **Culinary Uses:** Buckwheat is used to make soba noodles in Japanese cuisine. It's also ground into flour for pancakes, crepes, and gluten-free baking. Roasted buckwheat groats, known as kasha, are popular in Eastern European dishes.

Grain-like seeds such as quinoa, amaranth, and buckwheat offer exceptional nutritional benefits and culinary versatility. Their rich nutrient profiles, complete proteins, and gluten-free nature make them popular choices for various diets.

CHAPTER 4

Nutritional Value and Health Benefits

4.1 Macronutrient Breakdown

Macronutrient Breakdown in Nuts and Seeds:

1. Healthy Fats:

- **Monounsaturated and Polyunsaturated Fats:** Nuts and seeds are abundant sources of healthy fats, primarily monounsaturated and polyunsaturated fats. These include omega-3 and omega-6 fatty acids, essential for various bodily functions.

- **Benefits:** Healthy fats contribute to heart health by lowering LDL cholesterol, reducing inflammation, and supporting brain function.

2. Proteins:

- **Plant-Based Proteins:** Nuts and seeds are excellent sources of plant-based proteins, containing essential amino acids crucial for muscle repair, growth, and overall body function.

- **Benefits:** Protein aids in muscle development, supports immune function, and helps with satiety, aiding in weight management.

3. Carbohydrates:

- **Complex Carbohydrates:** Some nuts and seeds, especially quinoa and amaranth, contain complex carbohydrates that provide sustained energy and are high in dietary fiber.

- **Benefits:** Fiber aids digestion, regulates blood sugar levels, promotes a feeling of fullness, and supports overall gut health.

4. Dietary Fiber:

- **Soluble and Insoluble Fiber:** Nuts and seeds are rich in both types of dietary fiber, promoting digestive health and regular bowel movements.

- **Benefits:** Fiber helps in maintaining healthy cholesterol levels, regulates blood sugar, and supports a healthy gut microbiome.

5. Nutrient Density:

- **Vitamins and Minerals:** Nuts and seeds contain an array of vitamins (such as vitamin E, B vitamins, and vitamin K) and minerals (like magnesium, calcium, zinc, and iron), essential for various bodily functions.

- **Benefits:** These micronutrients play crucial roles in energy production, bone health, immune function, and overall well-being.

-

Nuts and seeds offer a well-rounded macronutrient profile, combining healthy fats, proteins, complex carbohydrates, dietary fiber, vitamins, and minerals. Incorporating these nutrient-dense foods into a balanced diet provides a host of health benefits, supporting heart health, aiding in digestion, managing blood sugar levels, promoting satiety, and contributing to overall well-being.

4.2 Micronutrients and Antioxidants

Micronutrients in Nuts and Seeds:

1. Vitamins:

- **Vitamin E:** Abundant in almonds, sunflower seeds, and hazelnuts, vitamin E acts as an antioxidant, protecting cells from damage caused by free radicals. It supports immune function and skin health.

- **B Vitamins:** Nuts and seeds contain various B vitamins, such as B1 (thiamine), B2 (riboflavin), B3 (niacin), B6, and folate. These play crucial roles in energy metabolism, nerve function, and red blood cell production.

- **Vitamin K:** Present in seeds like chia seeds, vitamin K is vital for blood clotting and bone health.

2. Minerals:

- **Magnesium:** Abundant in nuts like almonds and cashews, magnesium is crucial for nerve and muscle function, bone health, and regulating blood pressure.

- **Zinc:** Found in pumpkin seeds and cashews, zinc supports

immune function, wound
healing, and DNA synthesis.

- **Iron:** Some seeds, like
  pumpkin seeds and sunflower
  seeds, provide iron, which is
  essential for oxygen transport
  in the blood and overall energy
  production.

3. Antioxidants:

- **Polyphenols:** Present in
  various nuts and seeds,
  polyphenols act as antioxidants,
  protecting against cellular
  damage and inflammation.
  They contribute to heart health
  and may reduce the risk of
  chronic diseases.

- **Selenium:** Abundant in Brazil
  nuts, selenium is a powerful
  antioxidant that supports

immune function and thyroid
health.

**Health Benefits of Micronutrients
and Antioxidants:**

- **Cellular Protection:**
  Antioxidants in nuts and seeds
  help neutralize free radicals,
  reducing oxidative stress and
  lowering the risk of chronic
  diseases, including heart
  disease and certain cancers.

- **Immune Support:**
  Micronutrients like vitamin E,
  zinc, and selenium contribute to
  a robust immune system, aiding
  in fighting infections and
  supporting overall health.

- **Bone Health:** Vitamins like K
  and minerals like magnesium
  are crucial for bone health and

density, reducing the risk of osteoporosis.

- **Brain Health:** Certain antioxidants and B vitamins in nuts and seeds support cognitive function and may reduce the risk of age-related cognitive decline.

Nuts and seeds are packed with an impressive array of micronutrients and antioxidants that play critical roles in maintaining overall health. From supporting immune function to protecting against cellular damage and contributing to various bodily functions, these micronutrients and antioxidants make nuts and seeds not just tasty snacks but also nutritional powerhouses. Incorporating a variety of nuts and seeds into your diet can provide a rich source of these essential nutrients, contributing to a balanced and healthful lifestyle.

4.3 Health Benefits of Nuts and Seeds

The health benefits of nuts and seeds are numerous and diverse, ranging from heart health to improved brain function and overall well-being.

1. Heart Health:

- **Healthy Fats:** Nuts and seeds are rich in monounsaturated and polyunsaturated fats, which help lower LDL (bad) cholesterol levels, reducing the risk of heart disease and stroke.

- **Omega-3 Fatty Acids:** Certain seeds like flaxseeds and chia seeds, along with walnuts, contain omega-3 fatty acids that

support heart health by
reducing inflammation and
improving blood vessel
function.

- **Antioxidants:** Their high
antioxidant content, including
vitamin E and polyphenols,
helps prevent oxidative stress
and inflammation in the
arteries, promoting
cardiovascular health.

2. Weight Management:

- **Satiety:** Despite their calorie
density, the combination of
protein, healthy fats, and fiber
in nuts and seeds promotes a
feeling of fullness, potentially
reducing overall calorie intake
and aiding in weight
management.

- **Metabolism Support:** Some nuts, like almonds, have been associated with increased metabolism, potentially aiding in weight loss efforts.

3. Brain Function:

- **Omega-3s:** Omega-3 fatty acids found in certain seeds and nuts are crucial for brain health, supporting cognitive function, improving memory, and potentially reducing the risk of neurodegenerative diseases.

4. Diabetes Management:

- **Blood Sugar Regulation:** Nuts and seeds, especially those high in fiber like chia seeds and flaxseeds, can help regulate blood sugar levels, potentially benefiting individuals with diabetes.

5. Digestive Health:

- **Fiber Content:** The fiber in nuts and seeds supports digestive health by aiding regular bowel movements and maintaining a healthy gut microbiome.

6. Nutrient Density:

- **Vitamins and Minerals:** Nuts and seeds are dense in essential vitamins (like vitamin E, B vitamins) and minerals (such as magnesium, zinc, and iron), supporting various bodily functions and overall well-being.

7. Reduced Inflammation:

- **Antioxidants:** Their high content of antioxidants helps reduce inflammation throughout the body, potentially lowering the risk of chronic diseases associated with inflammation.

Incorporating nuts and seeds into a balanced diet offers a multitude of health benefits, from supporting heart health and brain function to aiding in weight management and promoting overall well-being. These nutrient-dense foods pack a powerful punch in terms of essential nutrients, healthy fats, antioxidants, and fiber, making them integral components of a health-conscious lifestyle.

4.4 Incorporating Nuts and Seeds into a Healthy Diet

Incorporating nuts and seeds into your diet is a flavorful and nutritious way to boost overall health. Here's how you can integrate them into your meals:

1. As Snacks:

- **Raw or Roasted:** Enjoy nuts like almonds, walnuts, or cashews as a quick and satisfying snack. Opt for unsalted varieties to control sodium intake.

- **Trail Mixes:** Create custom trail mixes by combining various nuts and seeds with dried fruits for a convenient, on-the-go snack.

2. Breakfast Options:

- **Sprinkle Over Cereals or Yogurt:** Add a crunchy texture by sprinkling chia seeds, flaxseeds, or sliced almonds over your morning cereal or yogurt.

- **Smoothie Boost:** Blend in a tablespoon of ground flaxseeds or chia seeds into your smoothies for an extra nutritional boost.

3. Salads and Soups:

- **Toppings:** Use toasted pumpkin seeds, sunflower seeds, or chopped nuts as toppings for salads or soups to add texture and flavor.

- **Homemade Dressings:** Incorporate nut or seed-based dressings or vinaigrettes for salads, enhancing both taste and nutrition.

4. Baking and Cooking:

- **Flour Alternatives:**
  Experiment with almond flour, flaxseed meal, or other nut/seed-based flours in baking for a nutritious alternative.

- **Crusts and Coatings:** Use crushed nuts or seeds as coatings for fish or poultry dishes, adding a delicious crunch.

5. Dips and Spreads:

- **Nut Butters:** Spread almond, peanut, or cashew butter on whole-grain toast or use them as a dip for fruits or veggies.

- **Seed-Based Dips:** Prepare hummus or pesto using sunflower or pumpkin seeds for a twist on traditional recipes.

6. Cooking Ingredients:

- **Stir-Fries and Curries:** Toss in cashews, peanuts, or sesame seeds into stir-fries or curries for added texture and flavor.

- **Quinoa and Grain Bowls:** Include quinoa, amaranth, or buckwheat as a base for grain bowls, topped with nuts or seeds for a well-rounded meal.

Tips for Incorporation:

- **Portion Control:** Nuts and seeds are nutrient-dense, so be mindful of portion sizes to manage calorie intake.

- **Diverse Selection:** Experiment with a variety of nuts and seeds to benefit from different nutritional profiles and flavors.

- **Whole Foods Preference:** Whenever possible, opt for

whole nuts and seeds rather
than processed versions to
maximize nutritional benefits.

Incorporating nuts and seeds into your
diet is versatile and delicious.
Whether used as snacks, toppings, or
cooking ingredients, they offer an
array of nutrients, healthy fats, and
flavors. By incorporating these
nutrient powerhouses into meals and
snacks, you can enhance the
nutritional value of your diet while
enjoying their diverse taste and
texture.

CHAPTER 5

Culinary Uses and Recipes

5.1 Cooking with Nuts and Seeds

5.1.1 Roasting Techniques:

- **Dry Roasting:** Spread nuts or seeds evenly on a baking sheet and roast in the oven at 350°F (175°C) for 8-15 minutes, stirring occasionally, until they turn golden and aromatic. This method works well for almonds, walnuts, and pumpkin seeds.

- **Stovetop Roasting:** Heat a dry skillet over medium heat, add nuts or seeds, and stir frequently until they're toasted to your desired level. Be attentive to prevent burning.

- **Flavor Variations:** Enhance roasted nuts by tossing them with spices like cinnamon, paprika, or a sprinkle of sea salt for savory or sweet variations.

5.1.2 Nut and Seed Butters:

- **Homemade Nut Butter:** Process roasted nuts or seeds in a food processor until they reach a creamy consistency. Add a pinch of salt or a drizzle of honey for flavor variation. Almonds, peanuts, and sunflower seeds work well for making butter.

- **Seed Butter Varieties:**
  Experiment with sesame seeds
  for tahini, pumpkin seeds for a
  nutty flavor, or sunflower seeds
  for a lighter taste.

5.1.3 Baking and Dessert Ideas:

- **Nuts in Baking:** Incorporate
  chopped nuts like almonds,
  walnuts, or pecans into muffins,
  cakes, cookies, or bread for
  added texture and flavor.

- **Seeds in Desserts:** Add chia
  seeds or flaxseeds to puddings,
  smoothies, or oatmeal for a
  nutritional boost and thicker
  consistency.

- **Energy Bars:** Create
  homemade energy bars using a
  mixture of nuts, seeds, dried
  fruits, oats, and a binder like

honey or nut butter. Press into a
pan and refrigerate until firm.

Recipes to Try:

1. Roasted Rosemary Almonds:

- **Ingredients:** Whole almonds,
  fresh rosemary, olive oil, sea
  salt.

- **Instructions:** Toss almonds
  with chopped rosemary, a
  drizzle of olive oil, and sea salt.
  Roast in the oven until golden
  brown and fragrant.

2. Homemade Peanut Butter:

- **Ingredients:** Roasted peanuts,
  a pinch of salt (optional).

- **Instructions:** Blend roasted
  peanuts in a food processor
  until creamy. Add salt if
  desired. Store in an airtight jar.

3. Chia Seed Pudding:

- **Ingredients:** Chia seeds, milk (dairy or plant-based), sweetener (honey, maple syrup), vanilla extract.

- **Instructions:** Mix chia seeds, milk, sweetener, and vanilla extract. Let it sit overnight in the fridge until it thickens, creating a pudding-like consistency.

Tips:

- **Storage:** Store nuts and seeds in airtight containers in a cool, dry place or the refrigerator to maintain freshness.

- **Experiment:** Don't be afraid to experiment with different nuts, seeds, and flavor combinations to discover your favorite culinary creations.

From roasting nuts for a crunchy snack to crafting homemade nut butters and incorporating seeds into baking and desserts, there are numerous ways to infuse your dishes with the goodness of nuts and seeds.

5.2 Recipes

5.2.1 Nutty Trail Mix:

- **Ingredients:**
    - 1 cup almonds
    - 1 cup cashews
    - 1 cup pumpkin seeds
    - 1 cup dried cranberries or raisins

- 1/2 cup dark chocolate chips or chunks (optional)

- 1/2 teaspoon cinnamon (optional)

- 1/4 teaspoon sea salt

- **Instructions:**

1.   Preheat the oven to 325°F (160°C).

2.   Mix almonds, cashews, and pumpkin seeds in a bowl. Add a sprinkle of cinnamon and sea salt.

3.   Spread the mixture evenly on a baking sheet and roast for 10-15 minutes until lightly golden.

4.   Let it cool completely, then add dried cranberries or raisins and chocolate chips if desired. Mix well and store in an airtight container.

5.2.2 Seed-Based Salad Dressings:

Creamy Tahini Dressing:

- **Ingredients:**

    - 1/4 cup tahini

    - 2 tablespoons olive oil

    - 2 tablespoons lemon juice

    - 1 clove garlic, minced

    - 2 tablespoons water

    - Salt and pepper to taste

- **Instructions:**

1.   Whisk together tahini, olive oil, lemon juice, minced garlic, and water in a bowl until smooth.

2.   Season with salt and pepper. Adjust consistency by adding more water if needed.

3.   Drizzle over salads or use as a dip for veggies.

5.2.3 Nut-Encrusted Protein Dishes:

Almond-Crusted Chicken:

- **Ingredients:**
  - 4 boneless, skinless chicken breasts
  - 1 cup almond meal
  - 1 teaspoon paprika
  - 1/2 teaspoon garlic powder
  - Salt and pepper to taste
  - 2 eggs, beaten
  - Olive oil for frying
- **Instructions:**

1.   Preheat the oven to 375°F (190°C). Grease a baking dish.

2.   In a bowl, mix almond meal, paprika, garlic powder, salt, and pepper.

3.   Dip each chicken breast in beaten eggs, then coat it with the almond meal mixture, pressing gently to adhere.

4.   Heat olive oil in a skillet over medium heat. Brown the chicken on both sides.

5.   Transfer the chicken to the prepared baking dish and bake for 20-25 minutes or until cooked through.

Tips:

- **Customization:** Feel free to personalize these recipes by adding your favorite nuts or seeds and adjusting flavors to suit your taste preferences.

- **Storage:** Store leftovers in airtight containers in the fridge to maintain freshness and flavor.

These recipes offer delicious ways to incorporate nuts and seeds into your meals. From a flavorful trail mix for on-the-go snacking to homemade salad dressings and nut-encrusted protein dishes, these recipes showcase the versatility and nutritional benefits of nuts and seeds, making your meals both tasty and nutritious!

CHAPTER 6

Allergies and Precautions

6.1 Common Nut and Seed Allergies

- **Tree Nuts:** Common tree nuts include almonds, walnuts, cashews, hazelnuts, pistachios, and Brazil nuts. Allergies to these nuts can be severe and potentially life-threatening.

- **Peanuts:** Despite being a legume, peanuts can cause allergic reactions similar to tree nuts and are one of the most common food allergens.

- **Seeds:** Sesame seeds, sunflower seeds, poppy seeds, and others can also trigger allergic reactions, although they're less common than tree nuts and peanuts.

6.2 Safety Measures and Cross-Contamination

- **Read Labels:** Always read food labels carefully to identify potential allergens. Manufacturers are required to highlight allergens in the ingredient list or as a separate statement (e.g., "Contains: peanuts, tree nuts").

- **Avoid Cross-Contamination:** When cooking or preparing meals, use separate utensils, cutting boards, and kitchen equipment to prevent cross-contact between nuts, seeds, and non-allergenic foods.

- **Ask at Restaurants:** When dining out, inquire about dishes and ask about potential nut or seed ingredients in the meals. Alert restaurant staff about your allergy.

- **Educate Others:** Inform friends, family, caregivers, and colleagues about your allergy, emphasizing the seriousness and potential consequences of exposure.

- **Emergency Plan:** Always carry prescribed medications like epinephrine (EpiPen) if you have a severe allergy. Be aware of the signs of an allergic reaction and how to use emergency medications.

Precautionary Measures:

- **Consult Medical Professionals:** Seek advice from allergists or healthcare providers to properly diagnose allergies and understand individual sensitivities.

- **Allergy Testing:** Undergo allergy testing to identify specific allergens, enabling better management and avoidance strategies.

- **Avoidance Strategies:** If allergic, consider avoiding products processed in facilities handling nuts or seeds to prevent accidental exposure.

Nut and seed allergies are serious and can lead to severe reactions. Individuals with allergies must take stringent precautions to avoid accidental exposure. Understanding allergens, reading labels, and practicing proper food handling can significantly reduce the risk of allergic reactions, allowing individuals to navigate their diets safely and responsibly. Always seek professional medical advice for proper diagnosis and management of allergies.

6.3 Alternative Options for Allergy-Sensitive Individuals

For individuals with nut or seed allergies, navigating food choices can be challenging. However, several alternative options exist to accommodate dietary needs and preferences:

1. Seed Alternatives:

- **Sunflower Seed Butter:** Substitute peanut or almond butter with sunflower seed butter as a spread or dip for a nut-free alternative.

- **Sesame Seed Paste (Tahini):** Use tahini in place of nut-based sauces or as a base for dressings, providing a creamy texture without nuts.

2. Non-Nut Flours:

- **Coconut Flour:** Replace almond flour or other nut flours with coconut flour in baking to avoid nut-based products.

- **Oat Flour:** Oat flour can be a suitable alternative in recipes that call for almond or hazelnut flour.

3. Protein Sources:

- **Beans and Legumes:** Utilize beans and legumes like chickpeas, lentils, and black beans as protein sources in meals.

- **Quinoa:** Opt for quinoa, a protein-rich pseudocereal, instead of nuts in salads, pilafs, or as a base for dishes.

4. Dairy-Free Milk:

- **Oat Milk, Rice Milk, or Hemp Milk:** Replace nut-based milk alternatives with options like oat, rice, or hemp

milk for beverages and
cooking.

5. Non-Nut Snacks:

- **Popcorn:** Choose air-popped
  popcorn seasoned with herbs or
  spices as a nut-free snack
  option.

- **Rice Cakes:** Enjoy rice cakes
  topped with spreads like
  hummus or seed-based butter
  for a satisfying snack.

6. Nut-Free Baking:

- **Seed Mixes:** Incorporate seed
  mixes like pumpkin, sunflower,
  chia, or flaxseeds into baking
  for added texture and
  nutritional benefits.

- **Banana or Applesauce:**
  Substitute mashed banana or
  applesauce for nuts in recipes

like muffins or cookies for moisture and flavor.

Precautionary Measures:

- **Read Labels:** Even with alternative options, always read labels to ensure products are free from nut or seed traces.

- **Cross-Contamination Awareness:** Be cautious of cross-contact in facilities handling allergens and look for products with allergy-friendly certifications.

Despite nut or seed allergies, a variety of alternative options exist to accommodate dietary needs. By exploring seed-based alternatives, non-nut flours, alternative protein sources, dairy-free milk, and nut-free snacks, individuals with allergies can still enjoy a diverse and flavorful diet.

Always practice caution, read labels attentively, and consult with allergists or healthcare providers to navigate food choices safely.

CHAPTER 7

Sustainability and Environmental Impact

The sustainability and environmental impact of nut and seed harvesting practices vary depending on several factors, including cultivation methods, water usage, land management, and transportation.

7.1 Harvesting Practices

1. Cultivation Methods:

- **Agroforestry:** Some nut trees, like almonds and walnuts, are often grown in agroforestry systems, promoting biodiversity by integrating trees with other crops or plants.

- **Mono-cropping vs. Polyculture:** Mono-cropping, where large expanses are dedicated to a single crop, can lead to soil depletion and increased vulnerability to pests. Polyculture, on the other hand, involves planting different crops together, enhancing biodiversity and soil health.

2. Water Usage:

- **Water-Intensive Crops:** Some nut crops, such as almonds, require substantial water resources. In regions facing water scarcity, extensive irrigation for nut cultivation can strain local water supplies.

- **Efficiency Measures:** Efforts to improve water efficiency through technologies like drip irrigation or utilizing water-saving techniques can mitigate environmental impact.

3. Land Management:

- **Sustainable Practices:** Implementing sustainable agricultural practices such as cover cropping, composting, and crop rotation helps maintain soil fertility and reduces the need for chemical fertilizers and pesticides.

- **Deforestation Concerns:** In some cases, large-scale nut and seed cultivation can contribute to deforestation, particularly in regions where forests are cleared to make way for plantations.

4. Transportation and Distribution:

- **Carbon Footprint:** The transportation of nuts and seeds from production areas to markets contributes to carbon emissions. Locally sourced or regionally grown nuts and seeds may have a lower carbon footprint compared to those imported from distant locations.

- **Packaging and Waste:** The packaging used for nuts and seeds, particularly single-use plastics, contributes to environmental waste. Efforts to use eco-friendly packaging materials and reduce waste are beneficial.

The sustainability of nut and seed harvesting practices depends on a range of factors, including cultivation methods, water usage, land management, and transportation. While some practices promote biodiversity, efficient water usage, and sustainable land management, others may contribute to environmental concerns such as water scarcity, deforestation, and carbon emissions. Efforts to adopt sustainable farming methods, conserve water, reduce carbon footprints in transportation, and minimize waste can contribute to a more environmentally friendly nut and seed industry.

7.2 Environmental Concerns

1. Water Usage:

- **High Water Demand:** Certain nut crops, like almonds and pistachios, require substantial water resources. In regions with water scarcity, excessive irrigation for these crops can strain local water supplies and ecosystems.

- **Impact on Aquifers and Rivers:** Intensive irrigation practices can lead to groundwater depletion and affect river systems, potentially harming aquatic ecosystems and wildlife dependent on these water sources.

2. Land Use and Deforestation:

- **Land Conversion:** Clearing forests or converting diverse landscapes into monoculture nut or seed plantations can lead to habitat loss, reducing biodiversity and disrupting local ecosystems.

- **Loss of Natural Habitats:** Large-scale production can contribute to the loss of natural habitats for various species, impacting biodiversity and ecological balance.

3. Chemical Usage:

- **Pesticides and Fertilizers:** Intensive nut and seed cultivation often involve the use of chemical pesticides and fertilizers, which can have adverse effects on soil health,

water quality, and surrounding
wildlife.

- **Runoff and Pollution:**
Chemical runoff from farms
can contaminate waterways,
causing pollution and harming
aquatic life.

4. Carbon Footprint:

- **Transportation Emissions:**
The transportation of nuts and
seeds over long distances
contributes to carbon
emissions, especially if they are
imported from distant locations.

- **Packaging Waste:** Single-use
plastic packaging and excessive
packaging contribute to
environmental waste and
pollution.

The production of nuts and seeds, while providing valuable nutritional resources, poses environmental challenges. Concerns such as excessive water usage, deforestation, chemical usage, and the carbon footprint of transportation are key areas that need attention within the industry. Adopting sustainable agricultural practices, efficient water management techniques, reduced chemical inputs, and mindful packaging and transportation strategies can mitigate these environmental concerns and contribute to a more environmentally friendly nut and seed industry.

7.3 Ethical Consumption of Nuts and Seeds

Ethical consumption of nuts and seeds involves considering the social and ethical implications of their production and consumption. Here are key aspects to consider:

1. Fair Labor Practices:

- **Worker Conditions:** Ensure that the farms or plantations where nuts and seeds are produced adhere to fair labor practices, providing safe working conditions and fair wages to workers.

- **Certifications:** Look for certifications like Fair Trade or Rainforest Alliance that support ethical labor practices and fair wages for farmers and workers.

2. Social Impact:

- **Community Benefits:** Support initiatives that benefit local communities in nut and seed production areas, such as community development projects or programs that improve access to education and healthcare.

3. Biodiversity and Conservation:

- **Support Sustainable Practices:** Choose products from producers that prioritize biodiversity conservation, avoiding practices that contribute to deforestation or habitat destruction.

4. Transparency and Accountability:

- **Traceability:** Opt for products with clear sourcing and transparent supply chains, ensuring that environmental and social standards are met throughout the production process.

- **Consumer Awareness:** Educate yourself and others about ethical issues related to nut and seed production, supporting companies that prioritize ethical sourcing and production.

5. Reduce Waste:

- **Sustainable Packaging:** Choose brands that use eco-friendly and minimal packaging to reduce waste and environmental impact.

6. Advocacy and Support:

- **Advocacy Initiatives:** Support organizations or initiatives that advocate for sustainable and ethical practices in the nut and seed industry.

Ethical consumption involves considering not just the nutritional benefits of nuts and seeds but also their social and environmental impact. By choosing products from sources that prioritize fair labor practices, environmental conservation, community development, and transparency in their supply chains, consumers can contribute to a more ethical and sustainable nut and seed industry. Being informed, supporting responsible brands, and advocating for ethical practices are essential steps towards promoting ethical consumption.

CHAPTER 8

Buying and Storing Guide

8.1 Selecting High-Quality Nuts and Seeds

1. Appearance:

- **Color and Texture:** Choose nuts and seeds that have vibrant coloration and a uniform appearance. Avoid those that appear discolored or have spots.

- **Texture:** Opt for nuts and seeds that are firm and not shriveled or soft, indicating freshness.

2. Smell:

- **Fresh Aroma:** High-quality nuts and seeds have a pleasant, nutty aroma. Avoid products with a rancid or stale smell, which might indicate spoilage.

3. Packaging:

- **Sealed Packaging:** Buy nuts and seeds from reputable brands or sources that package them in sealed containers or bags to ensure freshness.

4. Bulk Bins:

- **Check Freshness:** If buying from bulk bins, ensure that the nuts and seeds are frequently replenished to maintain freshness. Avoid bins where products look old or exposed to air for long periods.

8.2 Proper Storage Techniques

1. Cool and Dry:

- **Airtight Containers:** Transfer nuts and seeds to airtight containers or resealable bags to prevent exposure to air and moisture, which can lead to spoilage.

- **Cool Environment:** Store nuts and seeds in a cool, dark place away from heat and sunlight to maintain their quality. Consider using the refrigerator or freezer for longer-term storage.

2. Avoid Odor Absorption:

- **Separate Odorous Foods:** Keep nuts and seeds away from strong-smelling foods as they can absorb odors easily.

3. Freezing for Longevity:

- **Long-Term Storage:** For extended shelf life, especially for nuts, consider freezing them in airtight containers or freezer bags. This helps preserve freshness for several months.

4. Check Expiry Dates:

- **Stay Updated:** Check expiration dates on packaged nuts and seeds. Use them before the indicated date for the best quality.

5. Rotation:

- **First In, First Out (FIFO):** Use the oldest nuts and seeds first to maintain freshness. Rotate your stock to ensure you're consuming them before they lose their quality.

Selecting high-quality nuts and seeds involves examining their appearance, aroma, and packaging while ensuring they are fresh and well-packaged. Proper storage in airtight containers, away from heat and light, helps maintain their freshness. Freezing can extend their shelf life, and rotating your stock ensures you consume them before they degrade in quality.

8.3 Shelf Life and Preservation Tips

Shelf Life of Nuts:

- **Peanuts:** Stored properly, they can last for up to 1 year at room temperature and longer if refrigerated or frozen.

- **Almonds:** Kept in a cool, dry place, they can last around 1-2 years. Refrigeration or freezing can extend their shelf life to 2-3 years.

- **Walnuts:** Stored properly, they can last for about 1 year at room temperature. Refrigeration or freezing can extend their shelf life to 2-3 years.

- **Cashews:** Kept in a cool, dry place, they can last for around 1 year. Refrigeration or freezing can extend their shelf life to 2-3 years.

Shelf Life of Seeds:

- **Pumpkin Seeds:** Stored in a cool, dry place, they can last up to 1 year. Refrigeration or freezing can extend their shelf life to 2-3 years.

- **Sunflower Seeds:** Kept in a cool, dry place, they can last for about 1 year. Refrigeration or freezing can extend their shelf life to 2-3 years.

- **Chia Seeds:** Properly stored, they can last for around 2-4 years. Refrigeration or freezing can extend their shelf life to 4-5 years.

Preservation Tips:

- **Airtight Containers:** Use airtight containers or vacuum-sealed bags to store nuts and seeds, reducing exposure to air and moisture.

- **Refrigeration or Freezing:** For longer-term storage, especially in warmer climates, refrigerate or freeze nuts and seeds in sealed containers to maintain freshness.

- **Check for Rancidity:** Periodically check nuts and seeds for signs of rancidity, like an off smell or taste. Discard if they appear stale or have an unpleasant odor.

- **Rotate Stock:** Use the FIFO (First In, First Out) method to consume older nuts and seeds first to prevent spoilage.

- **Avoid Humidity:** Keep nuts and seeds away from humid environments to prevent mold growth.

The shelf life of nuts and seeds varies depending on storage conditions. Properly stored in cool, dry places or refrigerated/freezer environments, nuts and seeds can retain their quality

105

for extended periods. Airtight containers, proper rotation, and regular checks for freshness are key to preserving their taste and nutritional value. Following these preservation tips can help maximize the shelf life of nuts and seeds in your pantry.

Made in United States
Troutdale, OR
09/19/2024

22959348R00060